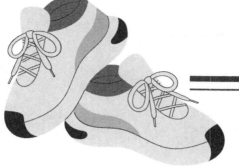

THIS BOOK BELONGS TO:

_____

_____

_____

_____

EMERGENCY CONTACT:

_____

_____

_____

_____

DATE: I'm feeling   ☺ ☺ ☹

Location:

Distance:

Pace:

Start Time: End Time:

Heart Rate:

Calories Burned:

Note:

DATE: I'm feeling   ☺ ☺ ☹

Location:

Distance:

Pace:

Start Time: End Time:

Heart Rate:

Calories Burned:

Note:

DATE: I'm feeling   ☺ ☺ ☹

Location:

Distance:

Pace:

Start Time: End Time:

Heart Rate:

Calories Burned:

Note:

DATE: I'm feeling   ☺ ☺ ☹

Location:

Distance:

Pace:

Start Time: End Time:

Heart Rate:

Calories Burned:

Note:

DATE: I'm feeling   ☺ ☹ ☹

Location:	
Distance:	
Pace:	
Start Time:	End Time:
Heart Rate:	
Calories Burned:	
Note:	

DATE: I'm feeling   ☺ ☹ ☹

Location:	
Distance:	
Pace:	
Start Time:	End Time:
Heart Rate:	
Calories Burned:	
Note:	

DATE: I'm feeling   ☺ ☹ ☹

Location:	
Distance:	
Pace:	
Start Time:	End Time:
Heart Rate:	
Calories Burned:	
Note:	

DATE: I'm feeling   ☺ ☹ ☹

Location:	
Distance:	
Pace:	
Start Time:	End Time:
Heart Rate:	
Calories Burned:	
Note:	

DATE:　　　　　　　　　　　　　　　　I'm feeling 　 ☺ 　😐 　☹

Location:

Distance:

Pace:

Start Time:　　　　　　　　　　　　　End Time:

Heart Rate:

Calories Burned:

Note:

DATE:　　　　　　　　　　　　　　　　I'm feeling 　 ☺ 　😐 　☹

Location:

Distance:

Pace:

Start Time:　　　　　　　　　　　　　End Time:

Heart Rate:

Calories Burned:

Note:

DATE:　　　　　　　　　　　　　　　　I'm feeling 　 ☺ 　😐 　☹

Location:

Distance:

Pace:

Start Time:　　　　　　　　　　　　　End Time:

Heart Rate:

Calories Burned:

Note:

DATE:　　　　　　　　　　　　　　　　I'm feeling 　 ☺ 　😐 　☹

Location:

Distance:

Pace:

Start Time:　　　　　　　　　　　　　End Time:

Heart Rate:

Calories Burned:

Note:

DATE: I'm feeling   :)   :| :(

Location:

Distance:

Pace:

Start Time: End Time:

Heart Rate:

Calories Burned:

Note:

DATE: I'm feeling   :)   :| :(

Location:

Distance:

Pace:

Start Time: End Time:

Heart Rate:

Calories Burned:

Note:

DATE: I'm feeling   :)   :| :(

Location:

Distance:

Pace:

Start Time: End Time:

Heart Rate:

Calories Burned:

Note:

DATE: I'm feeling   :)   :| :(

Location:

Distance:

Pace:

Start Time: End Time:

Heart Rate:

Calories Burned:

Note:

DATE:

I'm feeling ☺ ☺ ☹

Location:

Distance:

Pace:

Start Time: End Time:

Heart Rate:

Calories Burned:

Note:

DATE:

I'm feeling ☺ ☺ ☹

Location:

Distance:

Pace:

Start Time: End Time:

Heart Rate:

Calories Burned:

Note:

DATE:

I'm feeling ☺ ☺ ☹

Location:

Distance:

Pace:

Start Time: End Time:

Heart Rate:

Calories Burned:

Note:

DATE:

I'm feeling ☺ ☺ ☹

Location:

Distance:

Pace:

Start Time: End Time:

Heart Rate:

Calories Burned:

Note:

DATE:　　　　　　　　　　　　　I'm feeling　　😊　😐　☹️

Location:	
Distance:	
Pace:	
Start Time:	End Time:
Heart Rate:	
Calories Burned:	
Note:	

DATE:　　　　　　　　　　　　　I'm feeling　　😊　😐　☹️

Location:	
Distance:	
Pace:	
Start Time:	End Time:
Heart Rate:	
Calories Burned:	
Note:	

DATE:　　　　　　　　　　　　　I'm feeling　　😊　😐　☹️

Location:	
Distance:	
Pace:	
Start Time:	End Time:
Heart Rate:	
Calories Burned:	
Note:	

DATE:　　　　　　　　　　　　　I'm feeling　　😊　😐　☹️

Location:	
Distance:	
Pace:	
Start Time:	End Time:
Heart Rate:	
Calories Burned:	
Note:	

DATE: I'm feeling   ☺   😐   ☹

Location:
Distance:
Pace:
Start Time: End Time:
Heart Rate:
Calories Burned:
Note:

DATE: I'm feeling   ☺   😐   ☹

Location:
Distance:
Pace:
Start Time: End Time:
Heart Rate:
Calories Burned:
Note:

DATE: I'm feeling   ☺   😐   ☹

Location:
Distance:
Pace:
Start Time: End Time:
Heart Rate:
Calories Burned:
Note:

DATE: I'm feeling   ☺   😐   ☹

Location:
Distance:
Pace:
Start Time: End Time:
Heart Rate:
Calories Burned:
Note:

DATE: I'm feeling   ☺ ☺ ☹

Location:	
Distance:	
Pace:	
Start Time:	End Time:
Heart Rate:	
Calories Burned:	
Note:	

DATE: I'm feeling   ☺ ☺ ☹

Location:	
Distance:	
Pace:	
Start Time:	End Time:
Heart Rate:	
Calories Burned:	
Note:	

DATE: I'm feeling   ☺ ☺ ☹

Location:	
Distance:	
Pace:	
Start Time:	End Time:
Heart Rate:	
Calories Burned:	
Note:	

DATE: I'm feeling   ☺ ☺ ☹

Location:	
Distance:	
Pace:	
Start Time:	End Time:
Heart Rate:	
Calories Burned:	
Note:	

DATE: I'm feeling   ☺ 😐 ☹

Location:

Distance:

Pace:

Start Time: End Time:

Heart Rate:

Calories Burned:

Note:

DATE: I'm feeling   ☺ 😐 ☹

Location:

Distance:

Pace:

Start Time: End Time:

Heart Rate:

Calories Burned:

Note:

DATE: I'm feeling   ☺ 😐 ☹

Location:

Distance:

Pace:

Start Time: End Time:

Heart Rate:

Calories Burned:

Note:

DATE: I'm feeling   ☺ 😐 ☹

Location:

Distance:

Pace:

Start Time: End Time:

Heart Rate:

Calories Burned:

Note:

DATE:

I'm feeling ☺ 😐 ☹

Location:	
Distance:	
Pace:	
Start Time:	End Time:
Heart Rate:	
Calories Burned:	
Note:	

DATE:

I'm feeling ☺ 😐 ☹

Location:	
Distance:	
Pace:	
Start Time:	End Time:
Heart Rate:	
Calories Burned:	
Note:	

DATE:

I'm feeling ☺ 😐 ☹

Location:	
Distance:	
Pace:	
Start Time:	End Time:
Heart Rate:	
Calories Burned:	
Note:	

DATE:

I'm feeling ☺ 😐 ☹

Location:	
Distance:	
Pace:	
Start Time:	End Time:
Heart Rate:	
Calories Burned:	
Note:	

DATE: I'm feeling   ☺   😐   ☹

Location:

Distance:

Pace:

Start Time: End Time:

Heart Rate:

Calories Burned:

Note:

DATE: I'm feeling   ☺   😐   ☹

Location:

Distance:

Pace:

Start Time: End Time:

Heart Rate:

Calories Burned:

Note:

DATE: I'm feeling   ☺   😐   ☹

Location:

Distance:

Pace:

Start Time: End Time:

Heart Rate:

Calories Burned:

Note:

DATE: I'm feeling   ☺   😐   ☹

Location:

Distance:

Pace:

Start Time: End Time:

Heart Rate:

Calories Burned:

Note:

DATE: I'm feeling   :)   :| :(

Location:	
Distance:	
Pace:	
Start Time:	End Time:
Heart Rate:	
Calories Burned:	
Note:	

DATE: I'm feeling   :)   :| :(

Location:	
Distance:	
Pace:	
Start Time:	End Time:
Heart Rate:	
Calories Burned:	
Note:	

DATE: I'm feeling   :)   :| :(

Location:	
Distance:	
Pace:	
Start Time:	End Time:
Heart Rate:	
Calories Burned:	
Note:	

DATE: I'm feeling   :)   :| :(

Location:	
Distance:	
Pace:	
Start Time:	End Time:
Heart Rate:	
Calories Burned:	
Note:	

DATE: I'm feeling   ☺ ☺ ☹

| Location: |
| Distance: |
| Pace: |
| Start Time: | End Time: |
| Heart Rate: |
| Calories Burned: |
| Note: |

DATE: I'm feeling   ☺ ☺ ☹

| Location: |
| Distance: |
| Pace: |
| Start Time: | End Time: |
| Heart Rate: |
| Calories Burned: |
| Note: |

DATE: I'm feeling   ☺ ☺ ☹

| Location: |
| Distance: |
| Pace: |
| Start Time: | End Time: |
| Heart Rate: |
| Calories Burned: |
| Note: |

DATE: I'm feeling   ☺ ☺ ☹

| Location: |
| Distance: |
| Pace: |
| Start Time: | End Time: |
| Heart Rate: |
| Calories Burned: |
| Note: |

DATE: I'm feeling   ☺   😐   ☹

Location:	
Distance:	
Pace:	
Start Time:	End Time:
Heart Rate:	
Calories Burned:	
Note:	

DATE: I'm feeling   ☺   😐   ☹

Location:	
Distance:	
Pace:	
Start Time:	End Time:
Heart Rate:	
Calories Burned:	
Note:	

DATE: I'm feeling   ☺   😐   ☹

Location:	
Distance:	
Pace:	
Start Time:	End Time:
Heart Rate:	
Calories Burned:	
Note:	

DATE: I'm feeling   ☺   😐   ☹

Location:	
Distance:	
Pace:	
Start Time:	End Time:
Heart Rate:	
Calories Burned:	
Note:	

DATE: I'm feeling ☺ 😐 ☹

Location:

Distance:

Pace:

Start Time: End Time:

Heart Rate:

Calories Burned:

Note:

DATE: I'm feeling ☺ 😐 ☹

Location:

Distance:

Pace:

Start Time: End Time:

Heart Rate:

Calories Burned:

Note:

DATE: I'm feeling ☺ 😐 ☹

Location:

Distance:

Pace:

Start Time: End Time:

Heart Rate:

Calories Burned:

Note:

DATE: I'm feeling ☺ 😐 ☹

Location:

Distance:

Pace:

Start Time: End Time:

Heart Rate:

Calories Burned:

Note:

DATE: I'm feeling   :)   :| :(

Location:	
Distance:	
Pace:	
Start Time:	End Time:
Heart Rate:	
Calories Burned:	
Note:	

DATE: I'm feeling   :)   :| :(

Location:	
Distance:	
Pace:	
Start Time:	End Time:
Heart Rate:	
Calories Burned:	
Note:	

DATE: I'm feeling   :)   :| :(

Location:	
Distance:	
Pace:	
Start Time:	End Time:
Heart Rate:	
Calories Burned:	
Note:	

DATE: I'm feeling   :)   :| :(

Location:	
Distance:	
Pace:	
Start Time:	End Time:
Heart Rate:	
Calories Burned:	
Note:	

DATE: I'm feeling   ☺ 😐 ☹

Location:

Distance:

Pace:

Start Time: End Time:

Heart Rate:

Calories Burned:

Note:

DATE: I'm feeling   ☺ 😐 ☹

Location:

Distance:

Pace:

Start Time: End Time:

Heart Rate:

Calories Burned:

Note:

DATE: I'm feeling   ☺ 😐 ☹

Location:

Distance:

Pace:

Start Time: End Time:

Heart Rate:

Calories Burned:

Note:

DATE: I'm feeling   ☺ 😐 ☹

Location:

Distance:

Pace:

Start Time: End Time:

Heart Rate:

Calories Burned:

Note:

DATE: I'm feeling   🙂   😐   🙁

Location:

Distance:

Pace:

Start Time: End Time:

Heart Rate:

Calories Burned:

Note:

DATE: I'm feeling   🙂   😐   🙁

Location:

Distance:

Pace:

Start Time: End Time:

Heart Rate:

Calories Burned:

Note:

DATE: I'm feeling   🙂   😐   🙁

Location:

Distance:

Pace:

Start Time: End Time:

Heart Rate:

Calories Burned:

Note:

DATE: I'm feeling   🙂   😐   🙁

Location:

Distance:

Pace:

Start Time: End Time:

Heart Rate:

Calories Burned:

Note:

DATE: I'm feeling ☺ 😐 ☹

Location:	
Distance:	
Pace:	
Start Time:	End Time:
Heart Rate:	
Calories Burned:	
Note:	

DATE: I'm feeling ☺ 😐 ☹

Location:	
Distance:	
Pace:	
Start Time:	End Time:
Heart Rate:	
Calories Burned:	
Note:	

DATE: I'm feeling ☺ 😐 ☹

Location:	
Distance:	
Pace:	
Start Time:	End Time:
Heart Rate:	
Calories Burned:	
Note:	

DATE: I'm feeling ☺ 😐 ☹

Location:	
Distance:	
Pace:	
Start Time:	End Time:
Heart Rate:	
Calories Burned:	
Note:	

DATE: I'm feeling ☺ 😐 ☹

Location:	
Distance:	
Pace:	
Start Time:	End Time:
Heart Rate:	
Calories Burned:	
Note:	

DATE: I'm feeling ☺ 😐 ☹

Location:	
Distance:	
Pace:	
Start Time:	End Time:
Heart Rate:	
Calories Burned:	
Note:	

DATE: I'm feeling ☺ 😐 ☹

Location:	
Distance:	
Pace:	
Start Time:	End Time:
Heart Rate:	
Calories Burned:	
Note:	

DATE: I'm feeling ☺ 😐 ☹

Location:	
Distance:	
Pace:	
Start Time:	End Time:
Heart Rate:	
Calories Burned:	
Note:	

DATE: I'm feeling   ☺   😐   ☹

Location:

Distance:

Pace:

Start Time: End Time:

Heart Rate:

Calories Burned:

Note:

DATE: I'm feeling   ☺   😐   ☹

Location:

Distance:

Pace:

Start Time: End Time:

Heart Rate:

Calories Burned:

Note:

DATE: I'm feeling   ☺   😐   ☹

Location:

Distance:

Pace:

Start Time: End Time:

Heart Rate:

Calories Burned:

Note:

DATE: I'm feeling   ☺   😐   ☹

Location:

Distance:

Pace:

Start Time: End Time:

Heart Rate:

Calories Burned:

Note:

DATE:	I'm feeling	☺ ☻ ☹

Location:
Distance:
Pace:
Start Time:	End Time:
Heart Rate:
Calories Burned:
Note:

DATE:	I'm feeling	☺ ☻ ☹

Location:
Distance:
Pace:
Start Time:	End Time:
Heart Rate:
Calories Burned:
Note:

DATE:	I'm feeling	☺ ☻ ☹

Location:
Distance:
Pace:
Start Time:	End Time:
Heart Rate:
Calories Burned:
Note:

DATE:	I'm feeling	☺ ☻ ☹

Location:
Distance:
Pace:
Start Time:	End Time:
Heart Rate:
Calories Burned:
Note:

DATE: I'm feeling   ☺   😐   ☹

Location:

Distance:

Pace:

Start Time: End Time:

Heart Rate:

Calories Burned:

Note:

DATE: I'm feeling   ☺   😐   ☹

Location:

Distance:

Pace:

Start Time: End Time:

Heart Rate:

Calories Burned:

Note:

DATE: I'm feeling   ☺   😐   ☹

Location:

Distance:

Pace:

Start Time: End Time:

Heart Rate:

Calories Burned:

Note:

DATE: I'm feeling   ☺   😐   ☹

Location:

Distance:

Pace:

Start Time: End Time:

Heart Rate:

Calories Burned:

Note:

DATE: I'm feeling   ☺   😐   ☹

Location:

Distance:

Pace:

Start Time: End Time:

Heart Rate:

Calories Burned:

Note:

DATE: I'm feeling   ☺   😐   ☹

Location:

Distance:

Pace:

Start Time: End Time:

Heart Rate:

Calories Burned:

Note:

DATE: I'm feeling   ☺   😐   ☹

Location:

Distance:

Pace:

Start Time: End Time:

Heart Rate:

Calories Burned:

Note:

DATE: I'm feeling   ☺   😐   ☹

Location:

Distance:

Pace:

Start Time: End Time:

Heart Rate:

Calories Burned:

Note:

DATE: I'm feeling   ☺ ☺ ☹

| Location: |
| Distance: |
| Pace: |
| Start Time: | End Time: |
| Heart Rate: |
| Calories Burned: |
| Note: |
| |

DATE: I'm feeling   ☺ ☺ ☹

| Location: |
| Distance: |
| Pace: |
| Start Time: | End Time: |
| Heart Rate: |
| Calories Burned: |
| Note: |
| |

DATE: I'm feeling   ☺ ☺ ☹

| Location: |
| Distance: |
| Pace: |
| Start Time: | End Time: |
| Heart Rate: |
| Calories Burned: |
| Note: |
| |

DATE: I'm feeling   ☺ ☺ ☹

| Location: |
| Distance: |
| Pace: |
| Start Time: | End Time: |
| Heart Rate: |
| Calories Burned: |
| Note: |
| |

DATE: I'm feeling   🙂 😐 🙁

Location:	
Distance:	
Pace:	
Start Time:	End Time:
Heart Rate:	
Calories Burned:	
Note:	

DATE: I'm feeling   🙂 😐 🙁

Location:	
Distance:	
Pace:	
Start Time:	End Time:
Heart Rate:	
Calories Burned:	
Note:	

DATE: I'm feeling   🙂 😐 🙁

Location:	
Distance:	
Pace:	
Start Time:	End Time:
Heart Rate:	
Calories Burned:	
Note:	

DATE: I'm feeling   🙂 😐 🙁

Location:	
Distance:	
Pace:	
Start Time:	End Time:
Heart Rate:	
Calories Burned:	
Note:	

DATE: I'm feeling   ☺ 😐 ☹

Location:

Distance:

Pace:

Start Time: End Time:

Heart Rate:

Calories Burned:

Note:

DATE: I'm feeling   ☺ 😐 ☹

Location:

Distance:

Pace:

Start Time: End Time:

Heart Rate:

Calories Burned:

Note:

DATE: I'm feeling   ☺ 😐 ☹

Location:

Distance:

Pace:

Start Time: End Time:

Heart Rate:

Calories Burned:

Note:

DATE: I'm feeling   ☺ 😐 ☹

Location:

Distance:

Pace:

Start Time: End Time:

Heart Rate:

Calories Burned:

Note:

DATE:　　　　　　　　　　I'm feeling　　😊　😐　☹️

Location:	
Distance:	
Pace:	
Start Time:	End Time:
Heart Rate:	
Calories Burned:	
Note:	

DATE:　　　　　　　　　　I'm feeling　　😊　😐　☹️

Location:	
Distance:	
Pace:	
Start Time:	End Time:
Heart Rate:	
Calories Burned:	
Note:	

DATE:　　　　　　　　　　I'm feeling　　😊　😐　☹️

Location:	
Distance:	
Pace:	
Start Time:	End Time:
Heart Rate:	
Calories Burned:	
Note:	

DATE:　　　　　　　　　　I'm feeling　　😊　😐　☹️

Location:	
Distance:	
Pace:	
Start Time:	End Time:
Heart Rate:	
Calories Burned:	
Note:	

DATE: I'm feeling   ☺ ☺ ☹

Location:

Distance:

Pace:

Start Time: End Time:

Heart Rate:

Calories Burned:

Note:

DATE: I'm feeling   ☺ ☺ ☹

Location:

Distance:

Pace:

Start Time: End Time:

Heart Rate:

Calories Burned:

Note:

DATE: I'm feeling   ☺ ☺ ☹

Location:

Distance:

Pace:

Start Time: End Time:

Heart Rate:

Calories Burned:

Note:

DATE: I'm feeling   ☺ ☺ ☹

Location:

Distance:

Pace:

Start Time: End Time:

Heart Rate:

Calories Burned:

Note:

DATE: I'm feeling   ☺   😐   ☹

Location:

Distance:

Pace:

Start Time: End Time:

Heart Rate:

Calories Burned:

Note:

DATE: I'm feeling   ☺   😐   ☹

Location:

Distance:

Pace:

Start Time: End Time:

Heart Rate:

Calories Burned:

Note:

DATE: I'm feeling   ☺   😐   ☹

Location:

Distance:

Pace:

Start Time: End Time:

Heart Rate:

Calories Burned:

Note:

DATE: I'm feeling   ☺   😐   ☹

Location:

Distance:

Pace:

Start Time: End Time:

Heart Rate:

Calories Burned:

Note:

DATE:

I'm feeling 🙂 😐 🙁

Location:
Distance:
Pace:
Start Time: End Time:
Heart Rate:
Calories Burned:
Note:

DATE:

I'm feeling 🙂 😐 🙁

Location:
Distance:
Pace:
Start Time: End Time:
Heart Rate:
Calories Burned:
Note:

DATE:

I'm feeling 🙂 😐 🙁

Location:
Distance:
Pace:
Start Time: End Time:
Heart Rate:
Calories Burned:
Note:

DATE:

I'm feeling 🙂 😐 🙁

Location:
Distance:
Pace:
Start Time: End Time:
Heart Rate:
Calories Burned:
Note:

DATE: I'm feeling   🙂 😐 ☹️

Location:	
Distance:	
Pace:	
Start Time:	End Time:
Heart Rate:	
Calories Burned:	
Note:	

DATE: I'm feeling   🙂 😐 ☹️

Location:	
Distance:	
Pace:	
Start Time:	End Time:
Heart Rate:	
Calories Burned:	
Note:	

DATE: I'm feeling   🙂 😐 ☹️

Location:	
Distance:	
Pace:	
Start Time:	End Time:
Heart Rate:	
Calories Burned:	
Note:	

DATE: I'm feeling   🙂 😐 ☹️

Location:	
Distance:	
Pace:	
Start Time:	End Time:
Heart Rate:	
Calories Burned:	
Note:	

DATE: I'm feeling   ☺ 😐 ☹

Location:

Distance:

Pace:

Start Time: End Time:

Heart Rate:

Calories Burned:

Note:

DATE: I'm feeling   ☺ 😐 ☹

Location:

Distance:

Pace:

Start Time: End Time:

Heart Rate:

Calories Burned:

Note:

DATE: I'm feeling   ☺ 😐 ☹

Location:

Distance:

Pace:

Start Time: End Time:

Heart Rate:

Calories Burned:

Note:

DATE: I'm feeling   ☺ 😐 ☹

Location:

Distance:

Pace:

Start Time: End Time:

Heart Rate:

Calories Burned:

Note:

DATE: I'm feeling   ☺   😐   ☹

Location:	
Distance:	
Pace:	
Start Time:	End Time:
Heart Rate:	
Calories Burned:	
Note:	

DATE: I'm feeling   ☺   😐   ☹

Location:	
Distance:	
Pace:	
Start Time:	End Time:
Heart Rate:	
Calories Burned:	
Note:	

DATE: I'm feeling   ☺   😐   ☹

Location:	
Distance:	
Pace:	
Start Time:	End Time:
Heart Rate:	
Calories Burned:	
Note:	

DATE: I'm feeling   ☺   😐   ☹

Location:	
Distance:	
Pace:	
Start Time:	End Time:
Heart Rate:	
Calories Burned:	
Note:	

DATE: I'm feeling   🙂 😐 🙁

Location:

Distance:

Pace:

Start Time: End Time:

Heart Rate:

Calories Burned:

Note:

DATE: I'm feeling   🙂 😐 🙁

Location:

Distance:

Pace:

Start Time: End Time:

Heart Rate:

Calories Burned:

Note:

DATE: I'm feeling   🙂 😐 🙁

Location:

Distance:

Pace:

Start Time: End Time:

Heart Rate:

Calories Burned:

Note:

DATE: I'm feeling   🙂 😐 🙁

Location:

Distance:

Pace:

Start Time: End Time:

Heart Rate:

Calories Burned:

Note:

DATE: I'm feeling   ☺ ☺ ☹

| Location: |
| Distance: |
| Pace: |
| Start Time: | End Time: |
| Heart Rate: |
| Calories Burned: |
| Note: |

DATE: I'm feeling   ☺ ☺ ☹

| Location: |
| Distance: |
| Pace: |
| Start Time: | End Time: |
| Heart Rate: |
| Calories Burned: |
| Note: |

DATE: I'm feeling   ☺ ☺ ☹

| Location: |
| Distance: |
| Pace: |
| Start Time: | End Time: |
| Heart Rate: |
| Calories Burned: |
| Note: |

DATE: I'm feeling   ☺ ☺ ☹

| Location: |
| Distance: |
| Pace: |
| Start Time: | End Time: |
| Heart Rate: |
| Calories Burned: |
| Note: |

DATE: I'm feeling   :)   :| :(

Location:	
Distance:	
Pace:	
Start Time:	End Time:
Heart Rate:	
Calories Burned:	
Note:	

DATE: I'm feeling   :)   :| :(

Location:	
Distance:	
Pace:	
Start Time:	End Time:
Heart Rate:	
Calories Burned:	
Note:	

DATE: I'm feeling   :)   :| :(

Location:	
Distance:	
Pace:	
Start Time:	End Time:
Heart Rate:	
Calories Burned:	
Note:	

DATE: I'm feeling   :)   :| :(

Location:	
Distance:	
Pace:	
Start Time:	End Time:
Heart Rate:	
Calories Burned:	
Note:	

DATE:

I'm feeling 😊 😐 ☹️

Location:	
Distance:	
Pace:	
Start Time:	End Time:
Heart Rate:	
Calories Burned:	
Note:	

DATE:

I'm feeling 😊 😐 ☹️

Location:	
Distance:	
Pace:	
Start Time:	End Time:
Heart Rate:	
Calories Burned:	
Note:	

DATE:

I'm feeling 😊 😐 ☹️

Location:	
Distance:	
Pace:	
Start Time:	End Time:
Heart Rate:	
Calories Burned:	
Note:	

DATE:

I'm feeling 😊 😐 ☹️

Location:	
Distance:	
Pace:	
Start Time:	End Time:
Heart Rate:	
Calories Burned:	
Note:	

DATE: I'm feeling   ☺ 😐 ☹

Location:

Distance:

Pace:

Start Time: End Time:

Heart Rate:

Calories Burned:

Note:

DATE: I'm feeling   ☺ 😐 ☹

Location:

Distance:

Pace:

Start Time: End Time:

Heart Rate:

Calories Burned:

Note:

DATE: I'm feeling   ☺ 😐 ☹

Location:

Distance:

Pace:

Start Time: End Time:

Heart Rate:

Calories Burned:

Note:

DATE: I'm feeling   ☺ 😐 ☹

Location:

Distance:

Pace:

Start Time: End Time:

Heart Rate:

Calories Burned:

Note:

DATE: I'm feeling   ☺ ☺ ☹

Location:

Distance:

Pace:

Start Time: End Time:

Heart Rate:

Calories Burned:

Note:

DATE: I'm feeling   ☺ ☺ ☹

Location:

Distance:

Pace:

Start Time: End Time:

Heart Rate:

Calories Burned:

Note:

DATE: I'm feeling   ☺ ☺ ☹

Location:

Distance:

Pace:

Start Time: End Time:

Heart Rate:

Calories Burned:

Note:

DATE: I'm feeling   ☺ ☺ ☹

Location:

Distance:

Pace:

Start Time: End Time:

Heart Rate:

Calories Burned:

Note:

DATE: I'm feeling   ☺ 😐 ☹

Location:

Distance:

Pace:

Start Time: End Time:

Heart Rate:

Calories Burned:

Note:

DATE: I'm feeling   ☺ 😐 ☹

Location:

Distance:

Pace:

Start Time: End Time:

Heart Rate:

Calories Burned:

Note:

DATE: I'm feeling   ☺ 😐 ☹

Location:

Distance:

Pace:

Start Time: End Time:

Heart Rate:

Calories Burned:

Note:

DATE: I'm feeling   ☺ 😐 ☹

Location:

Distance:

Pace:

Start Time: End Time:

Heart Rate:

Calories Burned:

Note:

DATE: I'm feeling   ☺   😐   ☹

Location:	
Distance:	
Pace:	
Start Time:	End Time:
Heart Rate:	
Calories Burned:	
Note:	

DATE: I'm feeling   ☺   😐   ☹

Location:	
Distance:	
Pace:	
Start Time:	End Time:
Heart Rate:	
Calories Burned:	
Note:	

DATE: I'm feeling   ☺   😐   ☹

Location:	
Distance:	
Pace:	
Start Time:	End Time:
Heart Rate:	
Calories Burned:	
Note:	

DATE: I'm feeling   ☺   😐   ☹

Location:	
Distance:	
Pace:	
Start Time:	End Time:
Heart Rate:	
Calories Burned:	
Note:	

DATE: I'm feeling   ☺ 😐 ☹

Location:
Distance:
Pace:
Start Time: End Time:
Heart Rate:
Calories Burned:
Note:

DATE: I'm feeling   ☺ 😐 ☹

Location:
Distance:
Pace:
Start Time: End Time:
Heart Rate:
Calories Burned:
Note:

DATE: I'm feeling   ☺ 😐 ☹

Location:
Distance:
Pace:
Start Time: End Time:
Heart Rate:
Calories Burned:
Note:

DATE: I'm feeling   ☺ 😐 ☹

Location:
Distance:
Pace:
Start Time: End Time:
Heart Rate:
Calories Burned:
Note:

DATE: I'm feeling   ☺   😐   ☹

Location:

Distance:

Pace:

Start Time: End Time:

Heart Rate:

Calories Burned:

Note:

DATE: I'm feeling   ☺   😐   ☹

Location:

Distance:

Pace:

Start Time: End Time:

Heart Rate:

Calories Burned:

Note:

DATE: I'm feeling   ☺   😐   ☹

Location:

Distance:

Pace:

Start Time: End Time:

Heart Rate:

Calories Burned:

Note:

DATE: I'm feeling   ☺   😐   ☹

Location:

Distance:

Pace:

Start Time: End Time:

Heart Rate:

Calories Burned:

Note:

DATE: I'm feeling   ☺   😐   ☹

Location:

Distance:

Pace:

Start Time: End Time:

Heart Rate:

Calories Burned:

Note:

DATE: I'm feeling   ☺   😐   ☹

Location:

Distance:

Pace:

Start Time: End Time:

Heart Rate:

Calories Burned:

Note:

DATE: I'm feeling   ☺   😐   ☹

Location:

Distance:

Pace:

Start Time: End Time:

Heart Rate:

Calories Burned:

Note:

DATE: I'm feeling   ☺   😐   ☹

Location:

Distance:

Pace:

Start Time: End Time:

Heart Rate:

Calories Burned:

Note:

DATE: I'm feeling   ☺ 😐 ☹

Location:

Distance:

Pace:

Start Time: End Time:

Heart Rate:

Calories Burned:

Note:

DATE: I'm feeling   ☺ 😐 ☹

Location:

Distance:

Pace:

Start Time: End Time:

Heart Rate:

Calories Burned:

Note:

DATE: I'm feeling   ☺ 😐 ☹

Location:

Distance:

Pace:

Start Time: End Time:

Heart Rate:

Calories Burned:

Note:

DATE: I'm feeling   ☺ 😐 ☹

Location:

Distance:

Pace:

Start Time: End Time:

Heart Rate:

Calories Burned:

Note:

DATE: I'm feeling   ☺ 😐 ☹

Location:

Distance:

Pace:

Start Time: End Time:

Heart Rate:

Calories Burned:

Note:

DATE: I'm feeling   ☺ 😐 ☹

Location:

Distance:

Pace:

Start Time: End Time:

Heart Rate:

Calories Burned:

Note:

DATE: I'm feeling   ☺ 😐 ☹

Location:

Distance:

Pace:

Start Time: End Time:

Heart Rate:

Calories Burned:

Note:

DATE: I'm feeling   ☺ 😐 ☹

Location:

Distance:

Pace:

Start Time: End Time:

Heart Rate:

Calories Burned:

Note:

DATE: I'm feeling ☺ ☺ ☹

Location:	
Distance:	
Pace:	
Start Time:	End Time:
Heart Rate:	
Calories Burned:	
Note:	

DATE: I'm feeling ☺ ☺ ☹

Location:	
Distance:	
Pace:	
Start Time:	End Time:
Heart Rate:	
Calories Burned:	
Note:	

DATE: I'm feeling ☺ ☺ ☹

Location:	
Distance:	
Pace:	
Start Time:	End Time:
Heart Rate:	
Calories Burned:	
Note:	

DATE: I'm feeling ☺ ☺ ☹

Location:	
Distance:	
Pace:	
Start Time:	End Time:
Heart Rate:	
Calories Burned:	
Note:	

DATE: I'm feeling   ☺   😐   ☹

Location:

Distance:

Pace:

Start Time: End Time:

Heart Rate:

Calories Burned:

Note:

DATE: I'm feeling   ☺   😐   ☹

Location:

Distance:

Pace:

Start Time: End Time:

Heart Rate:

Calories Burned:

Note:

DATE: I'm feeling   ☺   😐   ☹

Location:

Distance:

Pace:

Start Time: End Time:

Heart Rate:

Calories Burned:

Note:

DATE: I'm feeling   ☺   😐   ☹

Location:

Distance:

Pace:

Start Time: End Time:

Heart Rate:

Calories Burned:

Note:

DATE: I'm feeling   ☺ 😐 ☹

Location:	
Distance:	
Pace:	
Start Time:	End Time:
Heart Rate:	
Calories Burned:	
Note:	

DATE: I'm feeling   ☺ 😐 ☹

Location:	
Distance:	
Pace:	
Start Time:	End Time:
Heart Rate:	
Calories Burned:	
Note:	

DATE: I'm feeling   ☺ 😐 ☹

Location:	
Distance:	
Pace:	
Start Time:	End Time:
Heart Rate:	
Calories Burned:	
Note:	

DATE: I'm feeling   ☺ 😐 ☹

Location:	
Distance:	
Pace:	
Start Time:	End Time:
Heart Rate:	
Calories Burned:	
Note:	

DATE:　　　　　　　　　　　　　　　I'm feeling　　😊　😐　☹️

Location:

Distance:

Pace:

Start Time:　　　　　　　　　　　　End Time:

Heart Rate:

Calories Burned:

Note:

DATE:　　　　　　　　　　　　　　　I'm feeling　　😊　😐　☹️

Location:

Distance:

Pace:

Start Time:　　　　　　　　　　　　End Time:

Heart Rate:

Calories Burned:

Note:

DATE:　　　　　　　　　　　　　　　I'm feeling　　😊　😐　☹️

Location:

Distance:

Pace:

Start Time:　　　　　　　　　　　　End Time:

Heart Rate:

Calories Burned:

Note:

DATE:　　　　　　　　　　　　　　　I'm feeling　　😊　😐　☹️

Location:

Distance:

Pace:

Start Time:　　　　　　　　　　　　End Time:

Heart Rate:

Calories Burned:

Note:

DATE: I'm feeling ☺ 😐 ☹

Location:
Distance:
Pace:
Start Time:	End Time:
Heart Rate:
Calories Burned:
Note:

DATE: I'm feeling ☺ 😐 ☹

Location:
Distance:
Pace:
Start Time:	End Time:
Heart Rate:
Calories Burned:
Note:

DATE: I'm feeling ☺ 😐 ☹

Location:
Distance:
Pace:
Start Time:	End Time:
Heart Rate:
Calories Burned:
Note:

DATE: I'm feeling ☺ 😐 ☹

Location:
Distance:
Pace:
Start Time:	End Time:
Heart Rate:
Calories Burned:
Note:

DATE: I'm feeling   ☺ 😐 ☹

Location:

Distance:

Pace:

Start Time: End Time:

Heart Rate:

Calories Burned:

Note:

DATE: I'm feeling   ☺ 😐 ☹

Location:

Distance:

Pace:

Start Time: End Time:

Heart Rate:

Calories Burned:

Note:

DATE: I'm feeling   ☺ 😐 ☹

Location:

Distance:

Pace:

Start Time: End Time:

Heart Rate:

Calories Burned:

Note:

DATE: I'm feeling   ☺ 😐 ☹

Location:

Distance:

Pace:

Start Time: End Time:

Heart Rate:

Calories Burned:

Note:

DATE:

I'm feeling   ☺ ☺ ☹

Location:
Distance:
Pace:
Start Time: End Time:
Heart Rate:
Calories Burned:
Note:

DATE:

I'm feeling   ☺ ☺ ☹

Location:
Distance:
Pace:
Start Time: End Time:
Heart Rate:
Calories Burned:
Note:

DATE:

I'm feeling   ☺ ☺ ☹

Location:
Distance:
Pace:
Start Time: End Time:
Heart Rate:
Calories Burned:
Note:

DATE:

I'm feeling   ☺ ☺ ☹

Location:
Distance:
Pace:
Start Time: End Time:
Heart Rate:
Calories Burned:
Note:

DATE: I'm feeling   ☺   😐   ☹

Location:

Distance:

Pace:

Start Time: End Time:

Heart Rate:

Calories Burned:

Note:

DATE: I'm feeling   ☺   😐   ☹

Location:

Distance:

Pace:

Start Time: End Time:

Heart Rate:

Calories Burned:

Note:

DATE: I'm feeling   ☺   😐   ☹

Location:

Distance:

Pace:

Start Time: End Time:

Heart Rate:

Calories Burned:

Note:

DATE: I'm feeling   ☺   😐   ☹

Location:

Distance:

Pace:

Start Time: End Time:

Heart Rate:

Calories Burned:

Note:

DATE: I'm feeling   ☺   😐   ☹

Location:

Distance:

Pace:

Start Time: End Time:

Heart Rate:

Calories Burned:

Note:

DATE: I'm feeling   ☺   😐   ☹

Location:

Distance:

Pace:

Start Time: End Time:

Heart Rate:

Calories Burned:

Note:

DATE: I'm feeling   ☺   😐   ☹

Location:

Distance:

Pace:

Start Time: End Time:

Heart Rate:

Calories Burned:

Note:

DATE: I'm feeling   ☺   😐   ☹

Location:

Distance:

Pace:

Start Time: End Time:

Heart Rate:

Calories Burned:

Note:

DATE: I'm feeling   ☺ 😐 ☹

Location:

Distance:

Pace:

Start Time: End Time:

Heart Rate:

Calories Burned:

Note:

DATE: I'm feeling   ☺ 😐 ☹

Location:

Distance:

Pace:

Start Time: End Time:

Heart Rate:

Calories Burned:

Note:

DATE: I'm feeling   ☺ 😐 ☹

Location:

Distance:

Pace:

Start Time: End Time:

Heart Rate:

Calories Burned:

Note:

DATE: I'm feeling   ☺ 😐 ☹

Location:

Distance:

Pace:

Start Time: End Time:

Heart Rate:

Calories Burned:

Note:

DATE: I'm feeling   ☺ ☺ ☹

Location:
Distance:
Pace:
Start Time: End Time:
Heart Rate:
Calories Burned:
Note:

DATE: I'm feeling   ☺ ☺ ☹

Location:
Distance:
Pace:
Start Time: End Time:
Heart Rate:
Calories Burned:
Note:

DATE: I'm feeling   ☺ ☺ ☹

Location:
Distance:
Pace:
Start Time: End Time:
Heart Rate:
Calories Burned:
Note:

DATE: I'm feeling   ☺ ☺ ☹

Location:
Distance:
Pace:
Start Time: End Time:
Heart Rate:
Calories Burned:
Note:

DATE: I'm feeling   🙂 😐 🙁

Location:

Distance:

Pace:

Start Time: End Time:

Heart Rate:

Calories Burned:

Note:

DATE: I'm feeling   🙂 😐 🙁

Location:

Distance:

Pace:

Start Time: End Time:

Heart Rate:

Calories Burned:

Note:

DATE: I'm feeling   🙂 😐 🙁

Location:

Distance:

Pace:

Start Time: End Time:

Heart Rate:

Calories Burned:

Note:

DATE: I'm feeling   🙂 😐 🙁

Location:

Distance:

Pace:

Start Time: End Time:

Heart Rate:

Calories Burned:

Note:

DATE:

I'm feeling ☺ 😐 ☹

Location:	
Distance:	
Pace:	
Start Time:	End Time:
Heart Rate:	
Calories Burned:	
Note:	

DATE:

I'm feeling ☺ 😐 ☹

Location:	
Distance:	
Pace:	
Start Time:	End Time:
Heart Rate:	
Calories Burned:	
Note:	

DATE:

I'm feeling ☺ 😐 ☹

Location:	
Distance:	
Pace:	
Start Time:	End Time:
Heart Rate:	
Calories Burned:	
Note:	

DATE:

I'm feeling ☺ 😐 ☹

Location:	
Distance:	
Pace:	
Start Time:	End Time:
Heart Rate:	
Calories Burned:	
Note:	

DATE:　　　　　　　　　　　I'm feeling　　😊　😐　☹️

Location:	
Distance:	
Pace:	
Start Time:	End Time:
Heart Rate:	
Calories Burned:	
Note:	

DATE:　　　　　　　　　　　I'm feeling　　😊　😐　☹️

Location:	
Distance:	
Pace:	
Start Time:	End Time:
Heart Rate:	
Calories Burned:	
Note:	

DATE:　　　　　　　　　　　I'm feeling　　😊　😐　☹️

Location:	
Distance:	
Pace:	
Start Time:	End Time:
Heart Rate:	
Calories Burned:	
Note:	

DATE:　　　　　　　　　　　I'm feeling　　😊　😐　☹️

Location:	
Distance:	
Pace:	
Start Time:	End Time:
Heart Rate:	
Calories Burned:	
Note:	

DATE: I'm feeling   🙂 😐 🙁

Location:	
Distance:	
Pace:	
Start Time:	End Time:
Heart Rate:	
Calories Burned:	
Note:	

DATE: I'm feeling   🙂 😐 🙁

Location:	
Distance:	
Pace:	
Start Time:	End Time:
Heart Rate:	
Calories Burned:	
Note:	

DATE: I'm feeling   🙂 😐 🙁

Location:	
Distance:	
Pace:	
Start Time:	End Time:
Heart Rate:	
Calories Burned:	
Note:	

DATE: I'm feeling   🙂 😐 🙁

Location:	
Distance:	
Pace:	
Start Time:	End Time:
Heart Rate:	
Calories Burned:	
Note:	

DATE: I'm feeling   ☺   😐   ☹

Location:

Distance:

Pace:

Start Time: End Time:

Heart Rate:

Calories Burned:

Note:

DATE: I'm feeling   ☺   😐   ☹

Location:

Distance:

Pace:

Start Time: End Time:

Heart Rate:

Calories Burned:

Note:

DATE: I'm feeling   ☺   😐   ☹

Location:

Distance:

Pace:

Start Time: End Time:

Heart Rate:

Calories Burned:

Note:

DATE: I'm feeling   ☺   😐   ☹

Location:

Distance:

Pace:

Start Time: End Time:

Heart Rate:

Calories Burned:

Note:

DATE: I'm feeling   🙂 😐 🙁

Location:	
Distance:	
Pace:	
Start Time:	End Time:
Heart Rate:	
Calories Burned:	
Note:	

DATE: I'm feeling   🙂 😐 🙁

Location:	
Distance:	
Pace:	
Start Time:	End Time:
Heart Rate:	
Calories Burned:	
Note:	

DATE: I'm feeling   🙂 😐 🙁

Location:	
Distance:	
Pace:	
Start Time:	End Time:
Heart Rate:	
Calories Burned:	
Note:	

DATE: I'm feeling   🙂 😐 🙁

Location:	
Distance:	
Pace:	
Start Time:	End Time:
Heart Rate:	
Calories Burned:	
Note:	

DATE: I'm feeling   ☺   😐   ☹

Location:

Distance:

Pace:

Start Time: End Time:

Heart Rate:

Calories Burned:

Note:

DATE: I'm feeling   ☺   😐   ☹

Location:

Distance:

Pace:

Start Time: End Time:

Heart Rate:

Calories Burned:

Note:

DATE: I'm feeling   ☺   😐   ☹

Location:

Distance:

Pace:

Start Time: End Time:

Heart Rate:

Calories Burned:

Note:

DATE: I'm feeling   ☺   😐   ☹

Location:

Distance:

Pace:

Start Time: End Time:

Heart Rate:

Calories Burned:

Note:

DATE: I'm feeling   ☺ 😐 ☹

Location:
Distance:
Pace:
Start Time:	End Time:
Heart Rate:
Calories Burned:
Note:

DATE: I'm feeling   ☺ 😐 ☹

Location:
Distance:
Pace:
Start Time:	End Time:
Heart Rate:
Calories Burned:
Note:

DATE: I'm feeling   ☺ 😐 ☹

Location:
Distance:
Pace:
Start Time:	End Time:
Heart Rate:
Calories Burned:
Note:

DATE: I'm feeling   ☺ 😐 ☹

Location:
Distance:
Pace:
Start Time:	End Time:
Heart Rate:
Calories Burned:
Note:

DATE:

I'm feeling ☺ 😐 ☹

Location:
Distance:
Pace:
Start Time: End Time:
Heart Rate:
Calories Burned:
Note:

DATE:

I'm feeling ☺ 😐 ☹

Location:
Distance:
Pace:
Start Time: End Time:
Heart Rate:
Calories Burned:
Note:

DATE:

I'm feeling ☺ 😐 ☹

Location:
Distance:
Pace:
Start Time: End Time:
Heart Rate:
Calories Burned:
Note:

DATE:

I'm feeling ☺ 😐 ☹

Location:
Distance:
Pace:
Start Time: End Time:
Heart Rate:
Calories Burned:
Note:

DATE: I'm feeling   ☺ 😐 ☹

Location:	
Distance:	
Pace:	
Start Time:	End Time:
Heart Rate:	
Calories Burned:	
Note:	

DATE: I'm feeling   ☺ 😐 ☹

Location:	
Distance:	
Pace:	
Start Time:	End Time:
Heart Rate:	
Calories Burned:	
Note:	

DATE: I'm feeling   ☺ 😐 ☹

Location:	
Distance:	
Pace:	
Start Time:	End Time:
Heart Rate:	
Calories Burned:	
Note:	

DATE: I'm feeling   ☺ 😐 ☹

Location:	
Distance:	
Pace:	
Start Time:	End Time:
Heart Rate:	
Calories Burned:	
Note:	

DATE: I'm feeling   ☺   😐   ☹

Location:

Distance:

Pace:

Start Time: End Time:

Heart Rate:

Calories Burned:

Note:

DATE: I'm feeling   ☺   😐   ☹

Location:

Distance:

Pace:

Start Time: End Time:

Heart Rate:

Calories Burned:

Note:

DATE: I'm feeling   ☺   😐   ☹

Location:

Distance:

Pace:

Start Time: End Time:

Heart Rate:

Calories Burned:

Note:

DATE: I'm feeling   ☺   😐   ☹

Location:

Distance:

Pace:

Start Time: End Time:

Heart Rate:

Calories Burned:

Note:

DATE: I'm feeling   ☺ ☺ ☹

| Location: |
| Distance: |
| Pace: |
| Start Time: | End Time: |
| Heart Rate: |
| Calories Burned: |
| Note: |

DATE: I'm feeling   ☺ ☺ ☹

| Location: |
| Distance: |
| Pace: |
| Start Time: | End Time: |
| Heart Rate: |
| Calories Burned: |
| Note: |

DATE: I'm feeling   ☺ ☺ ☹

| Location: |
| Distance: |
| Pace: |
| Start Time: | End Time: |
| Heart Rate: |
| Calories Burned: |
| Note: |

DATE: I'm feeling   ☺ ☺ ☹

| Location: |
| Distance: |
| Pace: |
| Start Time: | End Time: |
| Heart Rate: |
| Calories Burned: |
| Note: |

DATE: I'm feeling   ☺   😐   ☹

Location:

Distance:

Pace:

Start Time: End Time:

Heart Rate:

Calories Burned:

Note:

DATE: I'm feeling   ☺   😐   ☹

Location:

Distance:

Pace:

Start Time: End Time:

Heart Rate:

Calories Burned:

Note:

DATE: I'm feeling   ☺   😐   ☹

Location:

Distance:

Pace:

Start Time: End Time:

Heart Rate:

Calories Burned:

Note:

DATE: I'm feeling   ☺   😐   ☹

Location:

Distance:

Pace:

Start Time: End Time:

Heart Rate:

Calories Burned:

Note:

DATE:

I'm feeling ☺ 😐 ☹

Location:	
Distance:	
Pace:	
Start Time:	End Time:
Heart Rate:	
Calories Burned:	
Note:	

DATE:

I'm feeling ☺ 😐 ☹

Location:	
Distance:	
Pace:	
Start Time:	End Time:
Heart Rate:	
Calories Burned:	
Note:	

DATE:

I'm feeling ☺ 😐 ☹

Location:	
Distance:	
Pace:	
Start Time:	End Time:
Heart Rate:	
Calories Burned:	
Note:	

DATE:

I'm feeling ☺ 😐 ☹

Location:	
Distance:	
Pace:	
Start Time:	End Time:
Heart Rate:	
Calories Burned:	
Note:	

DATE: I'm feeling   ☺   😐   ☹

Location:

Distance:

Pace:

Start Time: End Time:

Heart Rate:

Calories Burned:

Note:

DATE: I'm feeling   ☺   😐   ☹

Location:

Distance:

Pace:

Start Time: End Time:

Heart Rate:

Calories Burned:

Note:

DATE: I'm feeling   ☺   😐   ☹

Location:

Distance:

Pace:

Start Time: End Time:

Heart Rate:

Calories Burned:

Note:

DATE: I'm feeling   ☺   😐   ☹

Location:

Distance:

Pace:

Start Time: End Time:

Heart Rate:

Calories Burned:

Note:

DATE: I'm feeling   ☺ ☺ ☹

Location:

Distance:

Pace:

Start Time: End Time:

Heart Rate:

Calories Burned:

Note:

DATE: I'm feeling   ☺ ☺ ☹

Location:

Distance:

Pace:

Start Time: End Time:

Heart Rate:

Calories Burned:

Note:

DATE: I'm feeling   ☺ ☺ ☹

Location:

Distance:

Pace:

Start Time: End Time:

Heart Rate:

Calories Burned:

Note:

DATE: I'm feeling   ☺ ☺ ☹

Location:

Distance:

Pace:

Start Time: End Time:

Heart Rate:

Calories Burned:

Note:

DATE: I'm feeling   ☺   😐   ☹

Location:

Distance:

Pace:

Start Time: End Time:

Heart Rate:

Calories Burned:

Note:

DATE: I'm feeling   ☺   😐   ☹

Location:

Distance:

Pace:

Start Time: End Time:

Heart Rate:

Calories Burned:

Note:

DATE: I'm feeling   ☺   😐   ☹

Location:

Distance:

Pace:

Start Time: End Time:

Heart Rate:

Calories Burned:

Note:

DATE: I'm feeling   ☺   😐   ☹

Location:

Distance:

Pace:

Start Time: End Time:

Heart Rate:

Calories Burned:

Note:

DATE: I'm feeling   ☺ ☺ ☹

| Location: |
| Distance: |
| Pace: |
| Start Time: | End Time: |
| Heart Rate: |
| Calories Burned: |
| Note: |

DATE: I'm feeling   ☺ ☺ ☹

| Location: |
| Distance: |
| Pace: |
| Start Time: | End Time: |
| Heart Rate: |
| Calories Burned: |
| Note: |

DATE: I'm feeling   ☺ ☺ ☹

| Location: |
| Distance: |
| Pace: |
| Start Time: | End Time: |
| Heart Rate: |
| Calories Burned: |
| Note: |

DATE: I'm feeling   ☺ ☺ ☹

| Location: |
| Distance: |
| Pace: |
| Start Time: | End Time: |
| Heart Rate: |
| Calories Burned: |
| Note: |

DATE: I'm feeling   🙂 😐 🙁

Location:

Distance:

Pace:

Start Time: End Time:

Heart Rate:

Calories Burned:

Note:

DATE: I'm feeling   🙂 😐 🙁

Location:

Distance:

Pace:

Start Time: End Time:

Heart Rate:

Calories Burned:

Note:

DATE: I'm feeling   🙂 😐 🙁

Location:

Distance:

Pace:

Start Time: End Time:

Heart Rate:

Calories Burned:

Note:

DATE: I'm feeling   🙂 😐 🙁

Location:

Distance:

Pace:

Start Time: End Time:

Heart Rate:

Calories Burned:

Note:

DATE: I'm feeling   ☺   😐   ☹

Location:

Distance:

Pace:

Start Time: End Time:

Heart Rate:

Calories Burned:

Note:

DATE: I'm feeling   ☺   😐   ☹

Location:

Distance:

Pace:

Start Time: End Time:

Heart Rate:

Calories Burned:

Note:

DATE: I'm feeling   ☺   😐   ☹

Location:

Distance:

Pace:

Start Time: End Time:

Heart Rate:

Calories Burned:

Note:

DATE: I'm feeling   ☺   😐   ☹

Location:

Distance:

Pace:

Start Time: End Time:

Heart Rate:

Calories Burned:

Note:

DATE: I'm feeling   ☺ 😐 ☹

| Location: |
| Distance: |
| Pace: |
| Start Time: | End Time: |
| Heart Rate: |
| Calories Burned: |
| Note: |

DATE: I'm feeling   ☺ 😐 ☹

| Location: |
| Distance: |
| Pace: |
| Start Time: | End Time: |
| Heart Rate: |
| Calories Burned: |
| Note: |

DATE: I'm feeling   ☺ 😐 ☹

| Location: |
| Distance: |
| Pace: |
| Start Time: | End Time: |
| Heart Rate: |
| Calories Burned: |
| Note: |

DATE: I'm feeling   ☺ 😐 ☹

| Location: |
| Distance: |
| Pace: |
| Start Time: | End Time: |
| Heart Rate: |
| Calories Burned: |
| Note: |

DATE: I'm feeling   ☺ ☺ ☹

Location:

Distance:

Pace:

Start Time: End Time:

Heart Rate:

Calories Burned:

Note:

DATE: I'm feeling   ☺ ☺ ☹

Location:

Distance:

Pace:

Start Time: End Time:

Heart Rate:

Calories Burned:

Note:

DATE: I'm feeling   ☺ ☺ ☹

Location:

Distance:

Pace:

Start Time: End Time:

Heart Rate:

Calories Burned:

Note:

DATE: I'm feeling   ☺ ☺ ☹

Location:

Distance:

Pace:

Start Time: End Time:

Heart Rate:

Calories Burned:

Note:

DATE: I'm feeling   ☺   😐   ☹

Location:

Distance:

Pace:

Start Time: End Time:

Heart Rate:

Calories Burned:

Note:

DATE: I'm feeling   ☺   😐   ☹

Location:

Distance:

Pace:

Start Time: End Time:

Heart Rate:

Calories Burned:

Note:

DATE: I'm feeling   ☺   😐   ☹

Location:

Distance:

Pace:

Start Time: End Time:

Heart Rate:

Calories Burned:

Note:

DATE: I'm feeling   ☺   😐   ☹

Location:

Distance:

Pace:

Start Time: End Time:

Heart Rate:

Calories Burned:

Note:

DATE: I'm feeling   ☺ 😐 ☹

| Location: |
| Distance: |
| Pace: |
| Start Time: | End Time: |
| Heart Rate: |
| Calories Burned: |
| Note: |
| |

DATE: I'm feeling   ☺ 😐 ☹

| Location: |
| Distance: |
| Pace: |
| Start Time: | End Time: |
| Heart Rate: |
| Calories Burned: |
| Note: |
| |

DATE: I'm feeling   ☺ 😐 ☹

| Location: |
| Distance: |
| Pace: |
| Start Time: | End Time: |
| Heart Rate: |
| Calories Burned: |
| Note: |
| |

DATE: I'm feeling   ☺ 😐 ☹

| Location: |
| Distance: |
| Pace: |
| Start Time: | End Time: |
| Heart Rate: |
| Calories Burned: |
| Note: |
| |

DATE: I'm feeling 🙂 😐 🙁

Location:

Distance:

Pace:

Start Time: End Time:

Heart Rate:

Calories Burned:

Note:

DATE: I'm feeling 🙂 😐 🙁

Location:

Distance:

Pace:

Start Time: End Time:

Heart Rate:

Calories Burned:

Note:

DATE: I'm feeling 🙂 😐 🙁

Location:

Distance:

Pace:

Start Time: End Time:

Heart Rate:

Calories Burned:

Note:

DATE: I'm feeling 🙂 😐 🙁

Location:

Distance:

Pace:

Start Time: End Time:

Heart Rate:

Calories Burned:

Note:

DATE: I'm feeling   ☺ 😐 ☹

Location:	
Distance:	
Pace:	
Start Time:	End Time:
Heart Rate:	
Calories Burned:	
Note:	

DATE: I'm feeling   ☺ 😐 ☹

Location:	
Distance:	
Pace:	
Start Time:	End Time:
Heart Rate:	
Calories Burned:	
Note:	

DATE: I'm feeling   ☺ 😐 ☹

Location:	
Distance:	
Pace:	
Start Time:	End Time:
Heart Rate:	
Calories Burned:	
Note:	

DATE: I'm feeling   ☺ 😐 ☹

Location:	
Distance:	
Pace:	
Start Time:	End Time:
Heart Rate:	
Calories Burned:	
Note:	

DATE: I'm feeling   ☺ 😐 ☹

Location:

Distance:

Pace:

Start Time: End Time:

Heart Rate:

Calories Burned:

Note:

DATE: I'm feeling   ☺ 😐 ☹

Location:

Distance:

Pace:

Start Time: End Time:

Heart Rate:

Calories Burned:

Note:

DATE: I'm feeling   ☺ 😐 ☹

Location:

Distance:

Pace:

Start Time: End Time:

Heart Rate:

Calories Burned:

Note:

DATE: I'm feeling   ☺ 😐 ☹

Location:

Distance:

Pace:

Start Time: End Time:

Heart Rate:

Calories Burned:

Note:

DATE: I'm feeling ☺ 😐 ☹

Location:	
Distance:	
Pace:	
Start Time:	End Time:
Heart Rate:	
Calories Burned:	
Note:	

DATE: I'm feeling ☺ 😐 ☹

Location:	
Distance:	
Pace:	
Start Time:	End Time:
Heart Rate:	
Calories Burned:	
Note:	

DATE: I'm feeling ☺ 😐 ☹

Location:	
Distance:	
Pace:	
Start Time:	End Time:
Heart Rate:	
Calories Burned:	
Note:	

DATE: I'm feeling ☺ 😐 ☹

Location:	
Distance:	
Pace:	
Start Time:	End Time:
Heart Rate:	
Calories Burned:	
Note:	

DATE: I'm feeling   ☺   😐   ☹

Location:

Distance:

Pace:

Start Time: End Time:

Heart Rate:

Calories Burned:

Note:

DATE: I'm feeling   ☺   😐   ☹

Location:

Distance:

Pace:

Start Time: End Time:

Heart Rate:

Calories Burned:

Note:

DATE: I'm feeling   ☺   😐   ☹

Location:

Distance:

Pace:

Start Time: End Time:

Heart Rate:

Calories Burned:

Note:

DATE: I'm feeling   ☺   😐   ☹

Location:

Distance:

Pace:

Start Time: End Time:

Heart Rate:

Calories Burned:

Note:

DATE:

I'm feeling   :) :| :(

Location:	
Distance:	
Pace:	
Start Time:	End Time:
Heart Rate:	
Calories Burned:	
Note:	

DATE:

I'm feeling   :) :| :(

Location:	
Distance:	
Pace:	
Start Time:	End Time:
Heart Rate:	
Calories Burned:	
Note:	

DATE:

I'm feeling   :) :| :(

Location:	
Distance:	
Pace:	
Start Time:	End Time:
Heart Rate:	
Calories Burned:	
Note:	

DATE:

I'm feeling   :) :| :(

Location:	
Distance:	
Pace:	
Start Time:	End Time:
Heart Rate:	
Calories Burned:	
Note:	

DATE: I'm feeling   ☺ ☺ ☹

Location:

Distance:

Pace:

Start Time: End Time:

Heart Rate:

Calories Burned:

Note:

DATE: I'm feeling   ☺ ☺ ☹

Location:

Distance:

Pace:

Start Time: End Time:

Heart Rate:

Calories Burned:

Note:

DATE: I'm feeling   ☺ ☺ ☹

Location:

Distance:

Pace:

Start Time: End Time:

Heart Rate:

Calories Burned:

Note:

DATE: I'm feeling   ☺ ☺ ☹

Location:

Distance:

Pace:

Start Time: End Time:

Heart Rate:

Calories Burned:

Note:

DATE:　　　　　　　　　　　　I'm feeling　　😊　😐　☹️

Location:

Distance:

Pace:

Start Time:　　　　　　　　　　　End Time:

Heart Rate:

Calories Burned:

Note:

DATE:　　　　　　　　　　　　I'm feeling　　😊　😐　☹️

Location:

Distance:

Pace:

Start Time:　　　　　　　　　　　End Time:

Heart Rate:

Calories Burned:

Note:

DATE:　　　　　　　　　　　　I'm feeling　　😊　😐　☹️

Location:

Distance:

Pace:

Start Time:　　　　　　　　　　　End Time:

Heart Rate:

Calories Burned:

Note:

DATE:　　　　　　　　　　　　I'm feeling　　😊　😐　☹️

Location:

Distance:

Pace:

Start Time:　　　　　　　　　　　End Time:

Heart Rate:

Calories Burned:

Note:

DATE: I'm feeling   ☺   😐   ☹

Location:

Distance:

Pace:

Start Time: End Time:

Heart Rate:

Calories Burned:

Note:

DATE: I'm feeling   ☺   😐   ☹

Location:

Distance:

Pace:

Start Time: End Time:

Heart Rate:

Calories Burned:

Note:

DATE: I'm feeling   ☺   😐   ☹

Location:

Distance:

Pace:

Start Time: End Time:

Heart Rate:

Calories Burned:

Note:

DATE: I'm feeling   ☺   😐   ☹

Location:

Distance:

Pace:

Start Time: End Time:

Heart Rate:

Calories Burned:

Note:

DATE: I'm feeling   🙂 😐 🙁

Location:

Distance:

Pace:

Start Time: End Time:

Heart Rate:

Calories Burned:

Note:

DATE: I'm feeling   🙂 😐 🙁

Location:

Distance:

Pace:

Start Time: End Time:

Heart Rate:

Calories Burned:

Note:

DATE: I'm feeling   🙂 😐 🙁

Location:

Distance:

Pace:

Start Time: End Time:

Heart Rate:

Calories Burned:

Note:

DATE: I'm feeling   🙂 😐 🙁

Location:

Distance:

Pace:

Start Time: End Time:

Heart Rate:

Calories Burned:

Note:

DATE: I'm feeling   😊 😐 ☹️

Location:

Distance:

Pace:

Start Time: End Time:

Heart Rate:

Calories Burned:

Note:

DATE: I'm feeling   😊 😐 ☹️

Location:

Distance:

Pace:

Start Time: End Time:

Heart Rate:

Calories Burned:

Note:

DATE: I'm feeling   😊 😐 ☹️

Location:

Distance:

Pace:

Start Time: End Time:

Heart Rate:

Calories Burned:

Note:

DATE: I'm feeling   😊 😐 ☹️

Location:

Distance:

Pace:

Start Time: End Time:

Heart Rate:

Calories Burned:

Note:

DATE: I'm feeling   ☺ ☺ ☹

Location:	
Distance:	
Pace:	
Start Time:	End Time:
Heart Rate:	
Calories Burned:	
Note:	

DATE: I'm feeling   ☺ ☺ ☹

Location:	
Distance:	
Pace:	
Start Time:	End Time:
Heart Rate:	
Calories Burned:	
Note:	

DATE: I'm feeling   ☺ ☺ ☹

Location:	
Distance:	
Pace:	
Start Time:	End Time:
Heart Rate:	
Calories Burned:	
Note:	

DATE: I'm feeling   ☺ ☺ ☹

Location:	
Distance:	
Pace:	
Start Time:	End Time:
Heart Rate:	
Calories Burned:	
Note:	

DATE: I'm feeling   :)   :| :(

Location:

Distance:

Pace:

Start Time: End Time:

Heart Rate:

Calories Burned:

Note:

DATE: I'm feeling   :)   :| :(

Location:

Distance:

Pace:

Start Time: End Time:

Heart Rate:

Calories Burned:

Note:

DATE: I'm feeling   :)   :| :(

Location:

Distance:

Pace:

Start Time: End Time:

Heart Rate:

Calories Burned:

Note:

DATE: I'm feeling   :)   :| :(

Location:

Distance:

Pace:

Start Time: End Time:

Heart Rate:

Calories Burned:

Note:

DATE: I'm feeling   ☺   😐   ☹

Location:	
Distance:	
Pace:	
Start Time:	End Time:
Heart Rate:	
Calories Burned:	
Note:	

DATE: I'm feeling   ☺   😐   ☹

Location:	
Distance:	
Pace:	
Start Time:	End Time:
Heart Rate:	
Calories Burned:	
Note:	

DATE: I'm feeling   ☺   😐   ☹

Location:	
Distance:	
Pace:	
Start Time:	End Time:
Heart Rate:	
Calories Burned:	
Note:	

DATE: I'm feeling   ☺   😐   ☹

Location:	
Distance:	
Pace:	
Start Time:	End Time:
Heart Rate:	
Calories Burned:	
Note:	

DATE: I'm feeling   ☺ 😐 ☹

Location:
Distance:
Pace:
Start Time:	End Time:
Heart Rate:
Calories Burned:
Note:

DATE: I'm feeling   ☺ 😐 ☹

Location:
Distance:
Pace:
Start Time:	End Time:
Heart Rate:
Calories Burned:
Note:

DATE: I'm feeling   ☺ 😐 ☹

Location:
Distance:
Pace:
Start Time:	End Time:
Heart Rate:
Calories Burned:
Note:

DATE: I'm feeling   ☺ 😐 ☹

Location:
Distance:
Pace:
Start Time:	End Time:
Heart Rate:
Calories Burned:
Note:

DATE: I'm feeling 🙂 😐 🙁

Location:

Distance:

Pace:

Start Time: End Time:

Heart Rate:

Calories Burned:

Note:

DATE: I'm feeling 🙂 😐 🙁

Location:

Distance:

Pace:

Start Time: End Time:

Heart Rate:

Calories Burned:

Note:

DATE: I'm feeling 🙂 😐 🙁

Location:

Distance:

Pace:

Start Time: End Time:

Heart Rate:

Calories Burned:

Note:

DATE: I'm feeling 🙂 😐 🙁

Location:

Distance:

Pace:

Start Time: End Time:

Heart Rate:

Calories Burned:

Note:

DATE: I'm feeling   ☺   😐   ☹

Location:

Distance:

Pace:

Start Time: End Time:

Heart Rate:

Calories Burned:

Note:

DATE: I'm feeling   ☺   😐   ☹

Location:

Distance:

Pace:

Start Time: End Time:

Heart Rate:

Calories Burned:

Note:

DATE: I'm feeling   ☺   😐   ☹

Location:

Distance:

Pace:

Start Time: End Time:

Heart Rate:

Calories Burned:

Note:

DATE: I'm feeling   ☺   😐   ☹

Location:

Distance:

Pace:

Start Time: End Time:

Heart Rate:

Calories Burned:

Note:

DATE: I'm feeling   ☺ ☺ ☹

Location:
Distance:
Pace:
Start Time: End Time:
Heart Rate:
Calories Burned:
Note:

DATE: I'm feeling   ☺ ☺ ☹

Location:
Distance:
Pace:
Start Time: End Time:
Heart Rate:
Calories Burned:
Note:

DATE: I'm feeling   ☺ ☺ ☹

Location:
Distance:
Pace:
Start Time: End Time:
Heart Rate:
Calories Burned:
Note:

DATE: I'm feeling   ☺ ☺ ☹

Location:
Distance:
Pace:
Start Time: End Time:
Heart Rate:
Calories Burned:
Note:

DATE: I'm feeling   ☺ 😐 ☹

Location:

Distance:

Pace:

Start Time: End Time:

Heart Rate:

Calories Burned:

Note:

DATE: I'm feeling   ☺ 😐 ☹

Location:

Distance:

Pace:

Start Time: End Time:

Heart Rate:

Calories Burned:

Note:

DATE: I'm feeling   ☺ 😐 ☹

Location:

Distance:

Pace:

Start Time: End Time:

Heart Rate:

Calories Burned:

Note:

DATE: I'm feeling   ☺ 😐 ☹

Location:

Distance:

Pace:

Start Time: End Time:

Heart Rate:

Calories Burned:

Note:

DATE: I'm feeling   😊 😐 ☹️

Location:	
Distance:	
Pace:	
Start Time:	End Time:
Heart Rate:	
Calories Burned:	
Note:	

DATE: I'm feeling   😊 😐 ☹️

Location:	
Distance:	
Pace:	
Start Time:	End Time:
Heart Rate:	
Calories Burned:	
Note:	

DATE: I'm feeling   😊 😐 ☹️

Location:	
Distance:	
Pace:	
Start Time:	End Time:
Heart Rate:	
Calories Burned:	
Note:	

DATE: I'm feeling   😊 😐 ☹️

Location:	
Distance:	
Pace:	
Start Time:	End Time:
Heart Rate:	
Calories Burned:	
Note:	

DATE: I'm feeling ☺ 😐 ☹

Location:	
Distance:	
Pace:	
Start Time:	End Time:
Heart Rate:	
Calories Burned:	
Note:	

DATE: I'm feeling ☺ 😐 ☹

Location:	
Distance:	
Pace:	
Start Time:	End Time:
Heart Rate:	
Calories Burned:	
Note:	

DATE: I'm feeling ☺ 😐 ☹

Location:	
Distance:	
Pace:	
Start Time:	End Time:
Heart Rate:	
Calories Burned:	
Note:	

DATE: I'm feeling ☺ 😐 ☹

Location:	
Distance:	
Pace:	
Start Time:	End Time:
Heart Rate:	
Calories Burned:	
Note:	

DATE: I'm feeling   🙂 😐 ☹️

Location:	
Distance:	
Pace:	
Start Time:	End Time:
Heart Rate:	
Calories Burned:	
Note:	

DATE: I'm feeling   🙂 😐 ☹️

Location:	
Distance:	
Pace:	
Start Time:	End Time:
Heart Rate:	
Calories Burned:	
Note:	

DATE: I'm feeling   🙂 😐 ☹️

Location:	
Distance:	
Pace:	
Start Time:	End Time:
Heart Rate:	
Calories Burned:	
Note:	

DATE: I'm feeling   🙂 😐 ☹️

Location:	
Distance:	
Pace:	
Start Time:	End Time:
Heart Rate:	
Calories Burned:	
Note:	

DATE: I'm feeling   :) :| :(

Location:

Distance:

Pace:

Start Time: End Time:

Heart Rate:

Calories Burned:

Note:

DATE: I'm feeling   :) :| :(

Location:

Distance:

Pace:

Start Time: End Time:

Heart Rate:

Calories Burned:

Note:

DATE: I'm feeling   :) :| :(

Location:

Distance:

Pace:

Start Time: End Time:

Heart Rate:

Calories Burned:

Note:

DATE: I'm feeling   :) :| :(

Location:

Distance:

Pace:

Start Time: End Time:

Heart Rate:

Calories Burned:

Note:

DATE: I'm feeling   ☺ ☺ ☹

Location:	
Distance:	
Pace:	
Start Time:	End Time:
Heart Rate:	
Calories Burned:	
Note:	

DATE: I'm feeling   ☺ ☺ ☹

Location:	
Distance:	
Pace:	
Start Time:	End Time:
Heart Rate:	
Calories Burned:	
Note:	

DATE: I'm feeling   ☺ ☺ ☹

Location:	
Distance:	
Pace:	
Start Time:	End Time:
Heart Rate:	
Calories Burned:	
Note:	

DATE: I'm feeling   ☺ ☺ ☹

Location:	
Distance:	
Pace:	
Start Time:	End Time:
Heart Rate:	
Calories Burned:	
Note:	

DATE: I'm feeling   ☺   😐   ☹

Location:

Distance:

Pace:

Start Time: End Time:

Heart Rate:

Calories Burned:

Note:

DATE: I'm feeling   ☺   😐   ☹

Location:

Distance:

Pace:

Start Time: End Time:

Heart Rate:

Calories Burned:

Note:

DATE: I'm feeling   ☺   😐   ☹

Location:

Distance:

Pace:

Start Time: End Time:

Heart Rate:

Calories Burned:

Note:

DATE: I'm feeling   ☺   😐   ☹

Location:

Distance:

Pace:

Start Time: End Time:

Heart Rate:

Calories Burned:

Note:

DATE: I'm feeling   ☺   😐   ☹

Location:
Distance:
Pace:
Start Time: End Time:
Heart Rate:
Calories Burned:
Note:

DATE: I'm feeling   ☺   😐   ☹

Location:
Distance:
Pace:
Start Time: End Time:
Heart Rate:
Calories Burned:
Note:

DATE: I'm feeling   ☺   😐   ☹

Location:
Distance:
Pace:
Start Time: End Time:
Heart Rate:
Calories Burned:
Note:

DATE: I'm feeling   ☺   😐   ☹

Location:
Distance:
Pace:
Start Time: End Time:
Heart Rate:
Calories Burned:
Note:

DATE:

I'm feeling 😊 😐 ☹️

Location:	
Distance:	
Pace:	
Start Time:	End Time:
Heart Rate:	
Calories Burned:	
Note:	

DATE:

I'm feeling 😊 😐 ☹️

Location:	
Distance:	
Pace:	
Start Time:	End Time:
Heart Rate:	
Calories Burned:	
Note:	

DATE:

I'm feeling 😊 😐 ☹️

Location:	
Distance:	
Pace:	
Start Time:	End Time:
Heart Rate:	
Calories Burned:	
Note:	

DATE:

I'm feeling 😊 😐 ☹️

Location:	
Distance:	
Pace:	
Start Time:	End Time:
Heart Rate:	
Calories Burned:	
Note:	

DATE: I'm feeling   ☺   😐   ☹

Location:

Distance:

Pace:

Start Time: End Time:

Heart Rate:

Calories Burned:

Note:

DATE: I'm feeling   ☺   😐   ☹

Location:

Distance:

Pace:

Start Time: End Time:

Heart Rate:

Calories Burned:

Note:

DATE: I'm feeling   ☺   😐   ☹

Location:

Distance:

Pace:

Start Time: End Time:

Heart Rate:

Calories Burned:

Note:

DATE: I'm feeling   ☺   😐   ☹

Location:

Distance:

Pace:

Start Time: End Time:

Heart Rate:

Calories Burned:

Note:

DATE: I'm feeling   ☺   😐   ☹

Location:

Distance:

Pace:

Start Time: End Time:

Heart Rate:

Calories Burned:

Note:

DATE: I'm feeling   ☺   😐   ☹

Location:

Distance:

Pace:

Start Time: End Time:

Heart Rate:

Calories Burned:

Note:

DATE: I'm feeling   ☺   😐   ☹

Location:

Distance:

Pace:

Start Time: End Time:

Heart Rate:

Calories Burned:

Note:

DATE: I'm feeling   ☺   😐   ☹

Location:

Distance:

Pace:

Start Time: End Time:

Heart Rate:

Calories Burned:

Note:

DATE:

I'm feeling   ☺ ☺ ☹

Location:	
Distance:	
Pace:	
Start Time:	End Time:
Heart Rate:	
Calories Burned:	
Note:	

DATE:

I'm feeling   ☺ ☺ ☹

Location:	
Distance:	
Pace:	
Start Time:	End Time:
Heart Rate:	
Calories Burned:	
Note:	

DATE:

I'm feeling   ☺ ☺ ☹

Location:	
Distance:	
Pace:	
Start Time:	End Time:
Heart Rate:	
Calories Burned:	
Note:	

DATE:

I'm feeling   ☺ ☺ ☹

Location:	
Distance:	
Pace:	
Start Time:	End Time:
Heart Rate:	
Calories Burned:	
Note:	

DATE: I'm feeling   :) :| :(

Location:

Distance:

Pace:

Start Time: End Time:

Heart Rate:

Calories Burned:

Note:

DATE: I'm feeling   :) :| :(

Location:

Distance:

Pace:

Start Time: End Time:

Heart Rate:

Calories Burned:

Note:

DATE: I'm feeling   :) :| :(

Location:

Distance:

Pace:

Start Time: End Time:

Heart Rate:

Calories Burned:

Note:

DATE: I'm feeling   :) :| :(

Location:

Distance:

Pace:

Start Time: End Time:

Heart Rate:

Calories Burned:

Note:

DATE: I'm feeling   ☺   ☹   ☹

Location:	
Distance:	
Pace:	
Start Time:	End Time:
Heart Rate:	
Calories Burned:	
Note:	

DATE: I'm feeling   ☺   ☹   ☹

Location:	
Distance:	
Pace:	
Start Time:	End Time:
Heart Rate:	
Calories Burned:	
Note:	

DATE: I'm feeling   ☺   ☹   ☹

Location:	
Distance:	
Pace:	
Start Time:	End Time:
Heart Rate:	
Calories Burned:	
Note:	

DATE: I'm feeling   ☺   ☹   ☹

Location:	
Distance:	
Pace:	
Start Time:	End Time:
Heart Rate:	
Calories Burned:	
Note:	

DATE:　　　　　　　　　　　　　　　I'm feeling　　☺　😐　☹

Location:	
Distance:	
Pace:	
Start Time:	End Time:
Heart Rate:	
Calories Burned:	
Note:	

DATE:　　　　　　　　　　　　　　　I'm feeling　　☺　😐　☹

Location:	
Distance:	
Pace:	
Start Time:	End Time:
Heart Rate:	
Calories Burned:	
Note:	

DATE:　　　　　　　　　　　　　　　I'm feeling　　☺　😐　☹

Location:	
Distance:	
Pace:	
Start Time:	End Time:
Heart Rate:	
Calories Burned:	
Note:	

DATE:　　　　　　　　　　　　　　　I'm feeling　　☺　😐　☹

Location:	
Distance:	
Pace:	
Start Time:	End Time:
Heart Rate:	
Calories Burned:	
Note:	

DATE: I'm feeling ☺ 😐 ☹

Location:	
Distance:	
Pace:	
Start Time:	End Time:
Heart Rate:	
Calories Burned:	
Note:	

DATE: I'm feeling ☺ 😐 ☹

Location:	
Distance:	
Pace:	
Start Time:	End Time:
Heart Rate:	
Calories Burned:	
Note:	

DATE: I'm feeling ☺ 😐 ☹

Location:	
Distance:	
Pace:	
Start Time:	End Time:
Heart Rate:	
Calories Burned:	
Note:	

DATE: I'm feeling ☺ 😐 ☹

Location:	
Distance:	
Pace:	
Start Time:	End Time:
Heart Rate:	
Calories Burned:	
Note:	

DATE: I'm feeling   🙂 😐 🙁

Location:

Distance:

Pace:

Start Time: End Time:

Heart Rate:

Calories Burned:

Note:

DATE: I'm feeling   🙂 😐 🙁

Location:

Distance:

Pace:

Start Time: End Time:

Heart Rate:

Calories Burned:

Note:

DATE: I'm feeling   🙂 😐 🙁

Location:

Distance:

Pace:

Start Time: End Time:

Heart Rate:

Calories Burned:

Note:

DATE: I'm feeling   🙂 😐 🙁

Location:

Distance:

Pace:

Start Time: End Time:

Heart Rate:

Calories Burned:

Note:

DATE: I'm feeling   ☺ 😐 ☹

Location:
Distance:
Pace:
Start Time:	End Time:
Heart Rate:
Calories Burned:
Note:

DATE: I'm feeling   ☺ 😐 ☹

Location:
Distance:
Pace:
Start Time:	End Time:
Heart Rate:
Calories Burned:
Note:

DATE: I'm feeling   ☺ 😐 ☹

Location:
Distance:
Pace:
Start Time:	End Time:
Heart Rate:
Calories Burned:
Note:

DATE: I'm feeling   ☺ 😐 ☹

Location:
Distance:
Pace:
Start Time:	End Time:
Heart Rate:
Calories Burned:
Note:

Printed in Great Britain
by Amazon

34659817R00069